Vegan Diet

For Beginners

The Ultimate Beginner's Vegan Diet Guide & Cookbook – Easy To Do Cookbook Recipes to Lose Weight and Stay Healthy + 30 Delicious Recipes

By Simone Jacobs

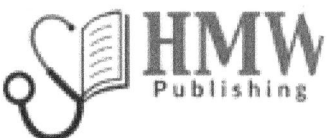

For more great books visit:

HMWPublishing.com

Get another book for Free

I want to thank you for purchasing this book and offer you another book (just as long and valuable as this book), "Health & Fitness Mistakes You Don't Know You're Making", completely free.

Visit the link below to signup and receive it:

www.hmwpublishing.com/gift

In this book, I will break down the most common health & fitness mistakes, you are probably committing right now, and I will reveal how you can easily get in the best shape of your life!

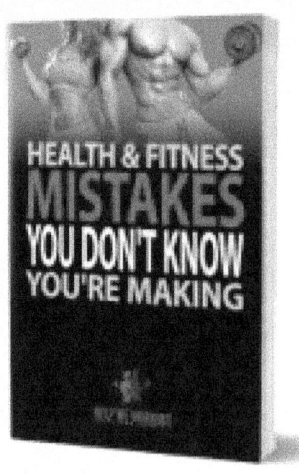

In addition to this valuable gift, you will also have an opportunity to get our new books for free, enter giveaways, and receive other valuable emails from me. Again, visit the link to sign up:

www.hmwpublishing.com/gift

TABLE OF CONTENTS

Introduction 1

Chapter 1: The Basics of Going Vegan 3

    Different Types of Vegan Diets 4
    Before You Make the Big Move 7
    What Truly is a Vegan Diet 12
    Getting the Vegan Myths Out of the Way 14

Chapter 2: The Health Benefits of a Vegan Diet 18

    Is It the Right Decision for You? 18
        Health 19
        Environment 20
        Ethical 21
    Going Vegan and Losing Weight 22
    Understanding Vegan Nutrition 22
        Fat. 23
        Omega 3 Fatty Acids 23
        Protein 24
        Vitamin D and Vitamin B12 25
        Calcium 25
        Other Minerals 26

Chapter 3: How to Transition to a Vegan Diet 29

    Transitioning Into Plant-based Foods 29
    Equipping Your Kitchen the Right Way 32
    Sticking to a Brand New Lifestyle 35

Chapter 4: Avoiding These Common Mistakes 38

    Avoiding the Risks of Veganism..........................38

    Writing Your Vegan Diet Plan.............................41

    Nutritional Features of Your Vegan Diet 44

        Caloric Macros (Macronutrients)....................44

Chapter 5: Vegan Breakfast Recipes 50

    Chive Waffles with Soy Mushrooms and Maple 50

    Avocado Salsa and Mexican Beans on Toast...53

    Lemon Poppy Scones 55

    Vegan Crepes..57

    Garbanzo-Oat Pancakes...................................59

Chapter 6: Vegan Lunch Recipes 61

    Seitan and Black Bean Stir-fry.........................61

    Eggless Tofu Spinach Quiche...........................64

    Vegan Mac and No Cheese...............................66

    Tomato, Basil, and Olive Oil Pasta 68

    Carrot Rice Nut Burger 70

Chapter 7: Vegan Dinner Recipes 72

    Sweet Potato and Coconut Curry.....................72

    Vegan Shepherd's Pie.......................................75

    Roast Summer Vegetables and Chickpeas 78

    Veggies and Tofu in Peanut Sauce...................80

    Vegan Fajitas..82

Chapter 8: Vegan Dessert Recipes 84

    Vegan Carrot Cake 84

Salted Caramel Biscuit Bar 88

Mint-Chip Coconut Milk Ice Cream 91

Orange Vegan Cake 93

Vegan Rose Meringues 95

Chapter 9: Vegan Soups, Stews and Salads .. 97

Crunchy Bulgur Salad 97

Tomato Soup 100

Barley and Lentil Stew 103

Spinach and Lentil Soup 105

Black Bean and Corn Salad 107

Chapter 10: Vegan Snack and Smoothie Recipe 109

Strawberry and Oatmeal Smoothie 109

Sweet Potato, Chili, and Peanut Butter Quesadillas 111

Raw Strawberry Jam 113

Vegan Cashew Cream Cheese 115

Kale and Banana Smoothie 117

Bonus Chapter: 14-Day Vegan Getting Started Plan 118

Final Words 123

About the Co-Author 124

Introduction

I want to thank you and congratulate you for purchasing the *"Vegan Diet for Beginners: The Ultimate Beginner's Vegan Guide & Cookbook."*

This book takes you on a spectacular journey with food and vegetables, specifically. If you do not already have a love affair with your friendly veggies, it is about time that you learn how to take advantage of the many benefits it offers. Veganism is not a fad it is a lifestyle—and you are getting the best guide through the whole journey, with this book. Thanks again for purchasing this book, I hope you enjoy reading it!

Also, before you get started, I recommend you **joining our email newsletter** to receive updates on any upcoming new book releases or promotions. You can sign-up for free, and as a bonus, you will receive a free gift. Our *"Health & Fitness Mistakes You Don't Know You're Making"* book! This book has been written to demystify, expose the top do's and don'ts and to finally equip you with the information you need to get in the best shape of your life. Due to the overwhelming amount of mis-information and lies told by magazines and self-proclaimed "gurus", it's becoming harder and harder to get reliable information to get in shape. As opposed to having to go through dozens of biased, unreliable and untrustworthy sources to get your health & fitness information. Everything you need to help you has been broken down in this book for you to easily follow and to immediately get results to achieve your desired fitness goals in the shortest amount of time.

Once again, to join our free email newsletter and to receive a free copy of this valuable book, please visit the link and signup now: **www.hmwpublishing.com/gift**

Chapter 1: The Basics of Going Vegan

Veganism is a specific diet that involves complete abstinence from all kinds of animal products. And those who decide to become vegan, do so because of the following reason:

1. Dietary Veganism. It is strict veganism, and when you follow this type of diet, you stay away from all kinds of animal products including dairy products and eggs. Anything that is an animal source should be avoided.

2. Ethical Veganism. It is a type of veganism that goes over and beyond the food restrictions because a person who is an ethical vegan will also abstain from the use of animals and animal products, for any purpose—like clothing.

3. Environmental Veganism. It is a type of veganism borne from the understanding that the means in which animal products are obtained is damaging to the environment.

Are you thinking of going vegan? Are you thinking of making the big leap but you are worried about a lot of things? In the next pages, you will discover enough to gain comfortable footing over the journey you are contemplating taking or gain even greater insights if you have already commited to be a vegan.

Different Types of Vegan Diets

You have looked into the common reasons why people decide to go Vegan. Here is a list of the different types of Vegan Diets. If you are exploring which direction to go, know that you can choose to be either one of these:

1. Ethical Vegan – As mentioned in the previous page, an ethical vegan is someone who abstains from the intake of all kinds of animals and animal by-products such as meat, cheese, honey, dairy, eggs, and fish. Aside from that, they do not wear clothing or accessories made from animals such as silk, leather, and fur; and they do not use cosmetic products tested on animals. Sometimes their moral stand goes over beyond consumption; as they can boycott a store that sells any animal products. Circuses and zoos are a disgrace to them; and their position as a vegan is born from their belief that all living beings are equal, so animals should not be exploited, in any way.

2. Plant Based Vegan – Many plant-based vegans decide to go vegan because of health reasons. Their diet is not very strict, and so they may consume honey or fish oil; and unlike ethical vegans, they may not refrain from the use of animal as clothing and so forth.

3. **Raw Vegan** – A person who chooses to become a raw vegan to embrace the health benefit it brings. Their diet is strict because apart from abstaining from animals or animal by-products, they do not consume anything that cooked above 115°F. Cooking usually depletes vegetables of their essential nutrients. A raw vegan's diet will be composed of vegetables, fruits, nuts, sprouts, seeds, roots, natural spices, fresh herbs, cold pressed oils, raw nut butters, raw nut milk, seaweeds, unprocessed olives, dried fruits, unpasteurized soy sauce, raw cocoa powder, vinegars, and pure maple syrup.

4. **Junk Food Vegan** – A junk food vegan is someone who is an ethical vegan, but is not at all concerned about the health benefits of going vegan. It means that they do not embrace the health feature of the diet, and may consume vegan junk food, quite excessively. It is proof that going vegan does not automatically mean that you are eating healthily.

Before You Make the Big Move

In whatever you do, it's nice to get the advice of experts. Especially if you are about to do something for the first time, and you have no clue about it, some tips will be of value.

Before the big move, here are some things you have to know:

1. Do not be in a hurry. The journey is not going to be easy, but it will be a fruitful one, especially when you complete it. Regardless of how big the mountain you have ahead of you, though, you should take your own pace. Try not to be in a hurry. Believe that you will get there, one-step-at-a-time. If you have to go one-animal-product-at-a-time, do it that way. If you want to start with one vegan meal a day, go ahead. The point is for you to get there—it doesn't matter how or how fast.

2. **Focus on the fruits and vegetables.** The big mistake people make about going vegan is they have too much of the starch products such as potatoes, pasta, rice, and bread. To compensate for the absence of meats, they fill up on starch which is rich in vitamins and nutrients like vegetables and fruits.

3. **Do not be afraid to experiment.** A lot of people think that vegans are malnourished, but that is not true. You should be more open about exploring the world of veganism so that you can maximize its full benefits. Play with tastes and open yourself up to new dishes, so that you can broaden your horizon.

4. **Choose whole grains.** Instead of having a lot of pasta and bread, choose whole grains, instead. They will also be a good source of protein, so make sure to pack on various types of grains.

5. Find the right support. People say that you get by with the help of friends and there is value in that, especially when you are a "baby" vegan. Working with a group is good because you become accountable to each other. You have someone to who will nag, remind, motivate, inspire, and guide you through it all. You can share experiences, tips, burdens, and so forth.

6. **Decide about how you acquire the food**. This may seem ridiculous, but it is crucial. Are you going to be cooking the food or are you going to pay for vegan food delivery? You have to realize that making the right food choices is going to be very difficult, so you need to be in complete control. By cooking your food you will know for sure what is on your plate—ordering from a vegan catering serving is good because it takes away the pressure from you, but you hardly have any choice about what gets delivered to your house. Still, these options will be easier compared to scouring a menu in a restaurant to see what fits into your diet.

7. **Declutter your life**. Rid yourself of old habits. Starting from the house, you have to clean your refrigerator and pantry to remove anything that goes against your new diet. Also, you have to make changes to your routine—less convenience store and fast food visits, unless you are sure that it fits in with your new lifestyle.

8. **Study the diet closely**. Eventually, you will get the hang of it, but as a newbie, you may feel completely lost. Before you begin, you have to give yourself some time to learn. This book is an excellent way to start because it will provide you with a rundown of all the stuff you have to know. Do not be content with knowing little. If you are going to do this, you have to do this right, so you need to study it. Your goal is to master the diet, even with your eyes closed. That way you can be confident that things won't go wrong.

9. **Be kind to yourself**. It will be hard, and you will have slip ups, but one or a few days should not define your journey so do not beat yourself up. If you fall, get back on the ride and keep on going. Do not be quick to abandon your journey—it will be worth it in the end.

10. **Learn how to supplement.** There are certain things that your diet may be lacking, such as iron, so you need to take supplements. You cannot deprive yourself of what it needs to function efficiently, so you look closely into your diet and determine what supplements you need to add.

What Truly is a Vegan Diet

There is a big question marks looming over the whole vegan phenomenon. People seem to be confused with the terms and inclusions, so if you are going to embark on this for real, you have to be fully aware.

The confusion is between Veganism and Vegetarianism. Vegetarians do not eat poultry, fish, and meat. Vegans are vegetarians who also do not eat or use dairy products, eggs, cosmetics, wool, silk, and soaps manufactured from animal products.

Based on the discussion earlier, one can choose to be vegan for a lot of reasons:

- Health
- Environment
- Ethics

Why do you want to be a vegan? The phenomenon of veganism can be traced back as early as 1944. However, it was in 1949 that Leslie J Cross gave its first definition: "The principle of the emancipation of animals from exploitation by man to seek an end to the use of animals by man for food, commodities, work, vivisection and by all other uses involving exploitation of animal by man."

This definition has evolved since, but, regarding food, a vegan's diet will be consist of vegetables, fruits, seeds, grains, nuts, pulses, and beans.

Getting the Vegan Myths Out of the Way

There are mixed reviews about the vegan diet, and if you are having doubts, it may be that you are concerned about some of the myths. Before you begin, it is necessary that you get these myths out of the way, to avoid the confusion. You have to understand veganism as a whole before you decide about it, so it's time for you to face the truth:

- "The food is bland and boring." People think vegan food has no character, but that is completely wrong. This book will give you fantastic 100% vegan recipes that are mouthwatering. There are so many ways to dress a bowl of vegetables if you know what to do. And about missing out on all the food, you are used to, understand that if you know where to look, there are vegan alternatives that will satisfy every craving you have.

- **"You will get frail and weak."** People have this thinking that the vegan diet is insufficient of everything necessary, so you will feel weak because your body is continually lacking. Do you know that many athletes maintain a strict vegan diet? A plant-based diet can sufficiently supply you with what you need, as long as you know how to do it right.

- **"It is not healthy."** In a nutshell, vegan is low-fat, and is a strict plant-based diet and is known to reverse and improve health conditions for people with heart disease and diabetes. It also prevents obesity, which is a rising problem, worldwide. How is that not healthy, at all? Still, vegan does not automatically mean it is healthy, mainly if you consume a lot of the vegan junk food. But ideally, the most simplistic form of this diet is very beneficial for your health.

- **"It is expensive to maintain."** Stick to the staples—bananas, potatoes, grains, and beans, because they are not just the healthiest, they are also the most convenient to have. If you know how to play with these ingredients, you will realize that the vegan diet is very cost-effective. And have you ever checked out how cheap vegetables are? It does not have to be wholefoods—you just have to know how to use the food that you can have.

- **"Eating out is going to be a nightmare."** People are so afraid to make the change to vegan because they think that eating out will be so difficult. If you know the vegan diet, through and through, you will realize that there are so many options for you. Also, there are more vegan places now, so it will not be so difficult. You can even ask the waiter for a vegan alternative to a dish you wish to order if you want to make things easier for yourself.

- "You will lack in protein." Since you are not eating meat, do you know where to source your protein from? Protein can be obtained from beans, nuts, pulses, and peas. You should not lack in protein if you include enough of these in your diet.

Chapter 2: The Health Benefits of a Vegan Diet

Just because you are taking on the vegan route doesn't mean you are the epitome of health. But the most carefully planned vegan diet can be very beneficial to your health and well-being.

Is It the Right Decision for You?

Why should you go vegan? Of the many diet disciplines around, why should you single out veganism? People choose to be vegan for three main things, their health, the environment, and for ethical reasons.

If you want to solidify your movement, you may want to understand the three aspects intimately:

Health

Regarding health, you make the turn to veganism and embrace the world of fruits and vegetables because you realize that they are your safest bets against all kinds of diseases:

- Cancer (Colon Cancer and Prostate Cancer)
- Cardiovascular Disease
- Hypertension
- Ischemic Heart Disease
- Obesity
- Stroke
- Type 2 Diabetes

The world is very toxic. There are a lot of potential poisons in the food world and when you finally realize the impact of this fact, know that you can make a turn to vegan and change your life. A well-constructed vegan meal plan can be very healthy. Your vegan lifestyle can very well prolong your life and improve the quality of life that you live.

Environment

Food is a necessity. Food production has become a priority, and it has been a big deal for a long time, but the world will be unable to sustain the agricultural impacts if it continues at the current rate. The demand for animal products has significantly risen through the years, so going vegan is also deciding to save the planet.

The practices involved in food production heavily exploit the planet's natural resources. If this goes on, conditions will get worse, and eventually, there would not be enough food to feed everyone.

You should understand that adopting a vegan lifestyle is going to result in less carbon footprint. So it is more than making a healthy choice for your body, you are also making a healthy turn for the planet (and everyone else in it).

Ethical

Have you given any thought to how the chicken on your plate got to your dinner table? The world has long enjoyed the consumption of meat while being oblivious to the awful truth involved in the slaughter of animals for food.

You do not have to be an animal lover to make this stand. But many of the known methods are very invasive, and the only way that you can actively take a move against these unhealthy practices is to refuse to support it. Your turn to veganism says to the world that you are the kind of person who will not sit and pretend it's okay to harm animals.

Those who choose to go vegan make this decision wholeheartedly, be it for their health, the environment, or animal welfare. Knowing what you know now, do you think this is the right decision for you?

Going Vegan and Losing Weight

Obesity is a leading world problem and a lot of lives are lost, every day, due to the ill-effects of obesity. Somehow, everything spirals down when you begin packing on extra pounds. Although being fit does not guarantee optimum health, obesity is not something you should be okay with.

Veganism and weight loss are mostly dependent on the high fiber content of vegetables and fruits. Fiber, if you do not know, is like a vacuum in your system. When you have a lot of fiber, your body will be more efficient at cleaning your digestive tract of toxins. Apart from its cleansing properties, vegetables are extremely low in calories so that it will help in weight control compared to another kind of diet.

Understanding Vegan Nutrition

So how can you maximize the full benefits of going vegan? It all sounds good on paper but how can you apply this lifestyle so that your body receives the right amount of nutrition it needs?

Fat

While you think you are being smart about missing out on the fat, by going vegan, the body still needs to be supplied with fat. To support this, you can source your fat from the following:

- Avocado
- Coconut
- Nut butter (cashew butter, peanut butter, walnut butter, almond butter, hazelnut butter)
- Nuts
- Oils (coconut oils, olive oil, avocado oil, canola oil, rice bran oil)
- Seed butter (pumpkin seed butter, sunflower butter, hemp seed butter)

Omega 3 Fatty Acids

A healthy kind of fat, you can get omega-3 fatty acids from canola oil, flaxseed, flaxseed oil, soybeans, tofu, and walnuts.

Protein

People think that protein is only sourced from animals and animal by-products. The body needs it because muscles and bones rely on it for healthy structure and repair. If you are going vegan, you will obtain your protein from:

- Almonds
- Broccoli
- Chickpeas
- Kale
- Lentils
- Peanut butter
- Peas
- Potatoes
- Rice
- Soy milk
- Spinach
- Tofu
- Whole wheat bread

Vitamin D and Vitamin B12

Vitamin D is not easily obtained in the vegan diet. B12, on the other hand, is scarce, but the demand is quite low. Regardless, you need to supply your diet accordingly. Of course, the most natural source of Vitamin D is still sunshine, but you can also obtain it from Vitamin D-fortified rice milk and soy milk. In the case of Vitamin B12, its vegan sources are:

- Red star nutritional yeast (vegetarian sports formula)
- Miso
- Seaweed
- Tempeh

Calcium

There is no doubt that the body needs calcium, zinc, iron and all kinds of minerals. Calcium is necessary for healthy bones, and they are obtained from the following sources:

- Almonds
- Blackstrap molasses
- Calcium-fortified soy milk
- Calcium-fortified orange juice
- Dark green vegetables
- Soybeans
- Soy yogurt
- Tahini
- Tofu

Other Minerals

Iron, which is necessary for blood health, is conveniently sourced from the following:

- Beet greens
- Black beans
- Black-eyed peas
- Blackstrap molasses
- Bokchoi
- Bulghur
- Chickpeas

- Kale
- Kidney beans
- Lentils
- Peas
- Prune juice
- Raisins
- Soybeans
- Swiss chard
- Tahini
- Tempeh
- Watermelon

Zinc is vital for pregnant women and is essential for the maintenance of the immune system. It may be sourced from:

- Legumes
- Nuts and seeds
- Grains
- Beans (kidney beans, garbanzo beans)

A good knowledge of food and their nutritional content is the key.

Chapter 3: How to Transition to a Vegan Diet

Transitioning from one diet to another is going to be a struggle. Abandoning old routines will not be easy, but a successful transition is truly impressive. In this chapter, you will learn how to take better control of your journey.

Transitioning Into Plant-based Foods

It seems simple, but you can ask anyone who has ever done it, and they will tell you that it is not. Making a change and adopting new habits can be very tricky, but it is not an impossibility.

The best way to tackle this is to follow a process. To make things simpler and more attainable, you will need a step-by-step plan of attack. For your journey to becoming a vegan, follow these steps to transition smoothly:

- **Step 1: Define your motivation.** Why are you making the transition? Are you doing this for health? Are you making an ethical choice for the environment and or for the welfare of animals? Do you want to lose weight? It is essential that this is clear because it will fuel your journey. If this is not adequately defined, it is quite easy to falter. But when there is a strong foundation established from the beginning, your transition will be backed up by a powerful motivation.

- **Step 2: Set your expectations.** It is not going to be a walk in the park. Whoever said it is going to be easy, probably did not go through the transition. It is tough, and you will want to quit, every time, so you have to be prepared. You have to be ready to be battling with yourself, the urges, the temptation, and so forth. Simply put, set your expectations realistically, but do not forget to remind yourself that it has been done before so you can do it too. Yes, it is hard, but there is a remarkable reward in the end.

- **Step 3: Educate yourself.** You cannot go through this without sitting down and studying it. The world of veganism is not something you do at a whim because there is so much to learn if you will do this right. It is more than just a knowledge of what to eat and what not to eat. This book sets you up at the right place, so take advantage of it.

- **Step 4: Write down a plan.** Armed with the right information, you can make things more attainable by writing down your ideas. It will serve as a guide so that you do not have to go through it like a headless chicken. A bonus chapter in this book includes a meal plan that you can use. It can be a template for the plan that you will write for yourself.

- **Step 5: Take it one day at a time.** Of course, all this physical and mental preparation will be for nothing without the corresponding action. If you are all set, then you have to make it happen. Just take it one day at a time. You do not have to hurry. If you fail one day, then you start all over again. Eventually, things will come naturally to you, and you will realize that veganism is already in your system.

Equipping Your Kitchen the Right Way

To launch your new lifestyle, you need to turn your kitchen into a vegan pantry. First you have to get rid of all the stuff that you do not need, throw it away or give it to someone; next you have to plan your meals; finally, you have to go shopping.

Shopping for food is going to be fun. As long as you know what to put into your shopping cart, it should not be so hard. As a beginner, you need to start with the basics. Eventually, you will build a vegan pantry that is fully-equipped.

Food	Sources
Butter Substitutes	oil and vegan butter
Carbohydrates	whole wheat pasta, soba noodles
Cheese Substitutes	nutritional yeast, rice cheese, soy cheese, nut and homemade vegan cheese
Condiments	Vegan mayonnaise, non-GMO mustard, and ketchup
Dairy Substitutes	almond yogurt, coconut yogurt, soy yogurt, vegan cream cheese
Egg Substitutes	applesauce and bananas, aquafaba, arrowroot eggs, chia seed eggs, chickpeas flour eggs, cornstarch eggs, ground flax seed eggs, tofu
Fruits	Any fruit in season especially those low in sugar such as grapefruit, lemon, cranberries, limes, pomegranate, strawberries, blueberries, blackcurrants
Milk Substitutes	almond milk, cashew milk, hemp milk, oat milk, rice milk, soy milk
Meat Substitutes	Field Roast sausages, Garden Fresh and Frozen Products, Sweet Earth

Nuts, Seeds and Dried Fruits	almonds, hemp seeds, chia seeds, ground flax seeds
Plant-Based Meat Substitutes	brown rice, bulgur, chickpeas, farro, legumes, organic non-GMO tofu, seitan, tempeh, quinoa, whole grains
Proteins	artichokes, asparagus, amaranth, almonds, beans, broccoli, black-eyed peas, chia seeds, chickpeas, edamame, green peas, green beans, hemp seeds, hemp milk, lentils, nutritional yeast, oatmeal, peanut butter, soy, spirulina, spinach, tahini, tofu, pumpkin seeds, quinoa
Seasonings	chili powder, cumin, dried basil, oregano, rosemary, and thyme, ground chipotle, ground ginger, onion powder, red pepper flakes, rice vinegar, sriracha, tamari or soy sauce,
Sweeteners	Blackstrap molasses, 100% organic maple syrup, unprocessed stevia, zulka

Vegetables	Anything in season. Leafy greens (most especially) But add a lot of parsley, garlic, cilantro, mint, and ginger (for flavoring)
Others	apple cider vinegar, chickpea flour, liquid smoke, olives, roasted red peppers, sundried tomatoes

Sticking to a Brand New Lifestyle

Once you successfully transition to veganism, your next goal is to maintain it. You have conquered the process, so it is necessary that you keep it in your system—otherwise, it will just be for nothing.

How can you stay vegan, now that you have already started? Here are some winning strategies you can apply:

- Keep your head in the game. Always remember your motivations and reasons, because it is supposed to give direction to your journey. If you want to keep going, you have to keep your head in the game.

- **Find joy in the eating vegan.** The mistake people make is they regard a diet like this as a "punishment." How can you find happiness, in punishment? You have to learn how to see the whole experience with a positive perspective. Explore the many amazing vegan recipes and allow yourself to enjoy the food selection. Healthy doesn't have to be boring. Vegan is not synonymous with bland. It can be magnificent.

- **Pack your food.** If dining out and going away is always a struggle for you, anticipate the worst. Instead of putting yourself in a wrong position, prepare for it. Pack your lunch to work, to trips, to meets, and so forth. Do not rely on the existence of a vegan menu. Instead, take matters into your own hands and pack your food.

- **Find healthy substitutes.** If you are afraid to indulge yourself with some of your cravings, then allow yourself tasty substitutes that will help bring happiness to your tummy.

- Transition slowly. Some people will consider going cold-turkey and abandon their old lifestyle to adopt an entirely vegan diet, but if you think this is going to be impossible, you can take it a pace that you can manage. Some people start by giving up on one animal product at a time until they become entirely vegan. You can begin with cutting on beef, or you can consider abandoning all meats except for seafood. Some people will start with one vegan meal per day until they are more confident about going completely vegan.

- Add exercise. If you want to give yourself room for some indulgence and you want to relax your diet, for a bit, add some physical activity that will keep things in control. This, in turn, will bring things in full circle because not only is your health consciousness focussed on the diet, but also the exercise.

Chapter 4: Avoiding These Common Mistakes

Your journey is not going to be an easy one, and you are bound to encounter problems along the way. Especially if you are not careful and you ignore the risks, things can go wrong.

As always, proper information is going to be your most potent weapon. If you take time to study veganism, it will be easier for you to avoid making mistakes.

Avoiding the Risks of Veganism

There are a few risks that you may encounter when you start the Vegan Diet:

1. **Eating too many calories.** Since rice, bread and noodles are non-animal, people tend to load up on these carbohydrates, so they end up eating so much more. As much as possible, concentrate on the vegetables and grains because they are the most nutritious. The mistake is that instead of becoming a vegetarian, one ends up being a starchatarian—and a diet like that is very high in calories.

2. **Eating too few calories.** Well, if you're not overeating, you may be eating too little. Vegetables are low in calorie, in general, and if your diet is concentrated on veggies, you may not supply your body efficiently. It, of course, will result in weakness and disease.

3. *Not getting enough nutrients.* You have to be realistic. Vegetables cannot solely sustain you, so you have to explore the world of veganism to be able to compensate your deficiency in protein, zinc, iron, calcium, Vitamin D, Vitamin B12 and omega-3 fatty acids. There are non-animal sources for these—and your knowledge is going to be important.

4. *Drinking an insufficient amount of water.* The body needs water (at least seven glasses a day), whether or not you are a vegan. But as one, water is necessary to move the fiber more efficiently. Your diet is going to be highly fibrous due to the fruits and vegetables, and you need water so that you can avoid problems with constipation, gas, and bloating.

5. **Putting little to no importance to meal planning.** Some people feel too confident, and so they abandon what they have been doing at the beginning of their journey, such as meal planning. That is fine really, but it makes you more prone to error. Meal planning allows you to be more exacting about your efforts. It guards your meals closely—so you can maintain the diet. As much as you can, religiously observe this habit so that you can check for nutrition, calories, and ingredients. Also, it is easier to ensure variety when you sit down to plan.

If you are not careful, it is easy to suffer from these risks, so make sure to pay more attention to what you are eating.

Writing Your Vegan Diet Plan

A sample plan is provided to you at the end of this book. You will use this plan as a template—so that you can begin to write your own. How do you write a diet plan?

- **Step 1: Know the boundaries of your diet.** What food can you eat? What food should you avoid? It is pertinent that you have laid down before anything else because the next steps will rely on your perfect knowledge of the boundaries of your diet.

- **Step 2: Determine your macro ratios and calories.** How many calories will you be taking in on a daily basis? Is this going to be sufficient for your primary and special needs? Are you going to be working out? If so, you have to make sure that your caloric intake supports this. What is the ratio of your caloric macronutrients? How much will protein, fat, and carbohydrates your diet have? It is essential that you determine this so that you can design a meal plan that satisfies your body's demands and requirements.

- **Step 3: How many meals are you going to have per day?** Are you going to have three meals—breakfast, lunch, and dinner; or will you be having five meals—breakfast, lunch, dinner, am and pm snacks? You need to decide on this because you have to divide the macronutrients and calories accordingly.

- **Step 4: Create your menu.** If you are an expert in the kitchen and writing your recipes, you can have fun in this section of your plan writing because this is where you stretch your imagination and creativity. If you are clueless about forming a recipe, do not worry because there are too many sources that you can use. This book has included as much as 30 recipes for you to try. Feel free to tweak them according to your taste.

- **Step 5: Start shopping.** You have written down everything and have carefully planned it; now it is time for you to write down a shopping list based on your meal plan. A meal plan is good because it directs your actions in the grocery or market. You do not have to go from aisle to aisle thinking of what to get; you just have to follow a list based on the plan. It's going to be easy.

Nutritional Features of Your Vegan Diet

This book has talked about calories, nutritional macros and so forth. Perhaps you are confused about how to plan your diet. The following is a guide that you can use:

Caloric Macros (Macronutrients)

A person's daily caloric intake depends on this requirement. A person may supply himself with 1500-3000 calories depending on how active he is.

Gender	Age	Calories		
		Sedentary	Moderately Active	Active
Child	2-3	1000	1000-1400	1000-1400
Male	4-8	1400	1400-1600	1600-2000
	9-13	1800	1800-2200	2000-2600
	14-18	2200	2400-2800	2800-3200
	19-30	2400	2600-2800	3000
	31-50+	2200	2400-2600	2800-3000
	51 above	2000	2200-2400	2400-2800

Female	4-8	1200	1400-1600	1400-1800
	9-13	1600	1600-2000	1800-2200
	14-18	1800	2000	2400
	19-30	2000	2000-2200	2400
	31-50	1800	2000	2200
	51+	1600	1800	2000-2200

Your caloric macros are consist of protein, fat, and carbohydrates. The percentage that each one will take will depend on your personal need. Those who engage in a lot of physical activity will need increased amounts of carbohydrates for energy; those who follow the ketogenic diet will maintain a high fat, low carb diet; and those who support the paleo diet will keep a high protein, low carb diet.

- Protein contains 4 calories per gram.
- Carbohydrates contain 4 calories per gram.

- Fat contains 9 calories per gram.

The table above shows you an estimate of how much calories you need per day, depending on how active your life is. The most common percentage split for these macronutrients is 40:40:20 where 20% is fat. You can change the percentage depending on the type of diet you want to have but use this equation to compute for calories:

daily calorie intake x macro percentage = calories

This means that if you follow the macro split given above, your fat requirement per day (if you are a 30-year-old-female with a sedentary lifestyle) will be:

$$2000 \times 0.2 = 400 \text{ calories}$$

Since there are 9 calories per gram of fat, 400 / 9 = 44.44 grams. You need 44.44 grams of fat per day.

Now, here is a rundown of your nutrient requirements. It is essential that you supply your diet accordingly, to satisfy your body's needs.

Nutrient	Daily Requirement
Protein	0.9 g per kg weight
Iron	14.4-32.4 mg
Calcium	1000 mg (men and women between 19-50 years)
Vitamin B12	2 mcg
Vitamin D	800 IU
Iodine	150-300 mg
Zinc	15 mg
Omega-3 Fatty Acids	250-500 mg

There are also some applications that you can download on your smartphone and gadgets to be able to do this efficiently. Applications like "MyFitnessPal" helps you take a record of your meals and activities per day while accounting for calories and nutrition. The use of these apps will help ensure that you are getting everything you need.

Have you enjoyed this book so far? Hopefully, you have learned so much because you're already halfway--the next chapters will be even more exciting.

Chapter 5: Vegan Breakfast Recipes

The first meal of the day is vital. A lot of people tend to neglect it, but it is a very wrong practice. Your breakfast is meant to jumpstart your day to a good light, so make sure to have a good meal in the morning.

Check out these easy-to-follow recipes:

Chive Waffles with Soy Mushrooms and Maple

Serves: 6

Preparation: 25 minutes

Cooking: 20 minutes

Ingredients:

- 1 tbsp baking powder
- 130g flour
- 1 tsp lemon juice

- 1 tbsp maple syrup
- 500ml rice milk or soya milk
- 6 mushrooms, sliced
- 150g polenta
- 2 tsp light soy sauce
- 100g sweet potato, mashed
- 2 tbsp rapeseed oil
- bunch of chives snipped
- olive oil
- soya yogurt (optional)
- salt and pepper, to taste

Directions:

1. In a bowl, combine the milk, rapeseed oil and vinegar. Mix them well and add the sweet potato mash and blend everything well.
2. In another bowl, combine the flour, polenta, and baking powder. Season with salt. Combine the contents of both bowls then add the chives to finish the batter.

3. Preheat the waffle iron, then pour batter and cook for about 4-5 minutes.
4. In a small bowl, combine soy sauce with maple syrup. Coat the mushrooms with this mixture then season it with pepper. Finally, saute the mushrooms until they are cooked through.
5. Serve the mushrooms on top of the waffles, then add a dollop of soya yogurt and a sprinkle of chives.

Calories	Fat	Carbohydrates	Fiber	Protein	Sodium
227	8g	30g	4g	7g	1.2g

Avocado Salsa and Mexican Beans on Toast

Serves: 4

Preparation: 20 minutes

Cooking: 10 minutes

Ingredients:

- 1 avocado, finely sliced
- 2 cans black beans
- 4 slices bread
- 1 tsp chili flakes or 2 tsp chipotle paste
- 1 tsp ground cumin
- 2 garlic cloves, crushed
- ½ lime, juiced
- 4 tbsp olive oil
- 1 onion, finely chopped
- 270g cherry tomatoes, quartered
- bunch of coriander

Directions:

1. In a bowl, combine lime juice, ¼ onion, tomatoes, and 1 tbsp oil then set it aside.
2. In a skillet, saute remaining onions and the garlic, then add the cumin and chili flakes (or chipotle). Add a splash of water and the beans, then add most of the tomato mixture with most of the coriander.
3. Meanwhile, toast the bread with a drizzle of the remaining ¼ oil.
4. To serve everything, lay a scoop of the bean mixture on the toast and add a few slices of avocado, and top it with the remaining coriander and tomato mixture.

Calories	Fat	Carbohydrates	Fiber	Protein	Sodium
368	19g	30g	13g	12g	0.9g

Lemon Poppy Scones

Serves: 12

Preparation: 10 minutes

Cooking 15 minutes

Ingredients:

- 4 tsp baking powder
- 2 cups all-purpose flour
- 1 lemon, juiced and zested
- ¾ cup margarine
- 2 tbsp poppy seeds
- ½ tsp salt
- ½ cup soy milk
- ¾ cup white sugar
- ½ cup water

1. Preheat on to 400°F. Grease a baking sheet.
2. In a bowl, combine flour, baking powder, sugar, salt and sift them all together. Slowly add the margarine until the mixture is smooth.

3. Add the lemon juice and zest, poppy seeds, soy milk, and water. Mix everything to form the batter.
4. Spoon ¼ cup sized batter onto the baking sheet and make sure they are about 3 inches apart from each other.
5. Pop them into the oven and bake them for about 10-15 minutes or until they are golden.

Calories	Fat	Carbohydrates	Protein	Sodium
250	12.3	30.8g	3 g	0.354g

Vegan Crepes

Serves: 4

Preparation: 5 minutes

Cooking: 20 minutes

Ingredients:

- 1 cup unbleached all-purpose flour
- 2 tbsp maple syrup
- ½ cup soy margarine
- ½ cup soy milk
- ¼ tsp salt
- 1 tbsp turbinado sugar
- ½ cup water

1. In a large bowl, combine water, soy milk, ¼ cup margarine, maple syrup, sugar, flour, and salt. Cover everything and chill it in the refrigerator for about 2 hours.

2. In a skillet, heat soy margarine and pour about 3 tbsp of batter to create the crepe. Flip it to cook the other side.
3. You can choose any fresh fruits for your filling.

Calories	Fat	Carbohydrates	Protein	Sodium
268	12.1g	35.6g	4.3g	0.295g

Garbanzo-Oat Pancakes

Serves: 4

Preparation: 5 minutes

Cooking: 15 minutes

Ingredients:

- 1 tsp baking powder
- ½ tsp ground cinnamon
- ¼ cup yellow cornmeal
- ½ cup garbanzo bean flour
- ¾ cup rolled oats
- 1 cup water

Directions:

1. In a large bowl, combine oats, garbanzo bean flour, cinnamon, cornmeal and baking powder. You may add more water if the mixture is too thick. Mix everything continuously until it is smooth and creamy.

2. In a griddle, heat oil and drop a large spoonful of the batter to cook it. Let it cook for about 3 minutes per side.
3. Serve the pancakes with your favorite fresh fruits or syrup.

Calories	Fat	Carbohydrates	Protein	Sodium
133	1.9g	24.5g	4.9	0.125g

Chapter 6: Vegan Lunch Recipes

Lunch serves as a pit stop meal, so if you have a very hectic day, this meal is going to be very important. This is essential in ensuring that the body is not going to run out of supply to perform its various functions.

Check out these easy-to-follow recipes:

Seitan and Black Bean Stir-fry

Serves: 4

Preparation: 20 minutes

Cooking: 25 minutes

Ingredients:

- 1 can black beans
- 1 red chili, finely chopped
- 1 tbsp cornflour
- 1 tsp Chinese five-spice powder

- 3 garlic cloves
- 2-3 tbsp vegetable oil
- 300g pak choi, chopped
- 1 tbsp peanut butter
- 2 tbsp rice vinegar
- 1 red pepper, sliced
- 1 jar seitan pieces
- 2 spring onions, sliced
- 75g brown sugar
- 2 tbsp soy sauce
- rice or noodles, cooked

Directions:

1. In a food processor, combine the beans with the brown sugar, garlic, soy sauce, five-spice powder, rice vinegar, peanut butter and red chili. Add water to make it smoother, then pour everything into a saucepan and heat it until it thickens.
2. Dry the seitan then toss them into a bowl with cornflour then set it aside.

3. In a large pan, heat oil then stir-fry the seitan until it is brown on the edges, then set it aside.
4. Using the same pan, dry it and add oil. Saute the peppers, pak choi, spring onion and the remaining beans. Add the seitan and pour in the sauce. Bring everything to a boil and serve it on top of the cooked rice or noodles.

Calories	Fat	Carbohydrates	Fiber	Protein	Sodium
326	8g	37g	7g	22g	3.08g

Eggless Tofu Spinach Quiche

Serves 6

Preparation: 15 minutes

Cooking: 30 minutes

Ingredients:

- 2/3 cup dairy-free cheddar cheese, shredded
- ½ cup dairy free Swiss cheese, shredded
- 1 tsp garlic, minced
- 1/3 cup almond milk
- ¼ cup onion, diced
- 9-inch unbaked pie crust
- 10 oz frozen spinach, thawed and chopped
- 8 oz tofu
- salt and pepper, to taste

Directions:

1. Preheat oven to 350°F
2. In a blender, combine milk and tofu then blend it until smooth. Season with salt and pepper.

3. In a bowl, combine garlic, spinach, onion, swiss cheese, cheddar cheese and the prepared tofu mixture. Mix everything well and then pour it into the pie crust
4. Pop it into the oven and let it bake for 30 minutes or until the top is golden brown.

Calories	Fat	Carbohydrates	Protein	Sodium
288	18.8g	18.5g	12.7g	0.489g

Vegan Mac and No Cheese

Serves: 4

Preparation: 15 minutes

Cooking 45 minutes

Ingredients:

- 1 cup cashews
- 1 tsp garlic powder
- 1/3 lemon juice
- 1 tsp onion powder
- 1 onion, chopped
- 8 oz elbow macaroni
- 1/3 cup canola oil
- 1 tbsp vegetable oil
- 4 oz roasted red peppers
- 1 1/3 cups water
- 3 tbsp nutritional yeast
- salt, to taste

Directions:

1. Preheat oven to 350°F
2. In a pot, boil water with a pinch of salt and cook the macaroni to al dente, for about 8 to 10 minutes. Set it aside in a baking dish.
3. In a saucepan, heat oil and saute onions until browned and then add this to the macaroni.
4. In a blender, combine lemon juice, cashews, water, and salt. Slowly add the roasted red peppers, canola oil, garlic powder, nutritional yeast and onion powder. Continue mixing everything until you achieve a smooth consistency.
5. Add the mixture to the macaroni and pop the dish into the oven to bake for about 10-15 minutes or until it has browned.

Calories	Fat	Carbohydrates	Fiber	Protein	Sodium
648	31.2g	69.6g	1g	16.5g	0.329g

Tomato, Basil, and Olive Oil Pasta

Serves: 8

Preparation: 15 minutes

Cooking 10 minutes

Ingredients:

- ½ cup fresh basil, cut into strips
- 2 cloves garlic, minced
- ½ cup olive oil
- 16 oz farfalle pasta
- 2 Roma tomatoes, seeded and diced
- salt and pepper, to taste

Directions:

1. In a pot, boil water with salt and cook the pasta to al dente, for 8 to 10 minutes. Drain and set it aside.
2. In a bowl, toss the cooked pasta with olive oil, tomatoes, basil, and garlic. Season with salt and pepper and serve.

Calories	Fat	Carbohydrates	Protein	Sodium
345	14.9g	44.1g	8.4g	3g

Carrot Rice Nut Burger

Serves: 20

Preparation: 1 hour

Cooking: 1 hour 30 minutes

Ingredients:

- 1 cup cashews, toasted
- 6 carrots, chopped
- 1 tbsp extra virgin olive oil
- 1 sweet onion, chopped
- 3 cups brown rice, uncooked
- 1 lb unsalted sunflower seeds, toasted
- 6 cups water
- salt, to taste

Directions:

1. In a pot, boil rice in water and reduce heat to let it simmer for about 45 minutes
2. In a food processor, combine cashews, sunflower seeds and let it run until smooth. Set it aside.

3. Run the onions and carrots in the food processor until finely shredded and combine it with the nuts.
4. Run the rice with oil in the food processor until smooth and mix this with everything. Season with salt and form patties.
5. Grill the patties about 6-8 minutes per side or until they are browned. Serve with whole-wheat buns or salad greens.

Calories	Fat	Carbohydrates	Protein	Sodium
270	16.2g	26.3g	7.7g	0.073g

Chapter 7: Vegan Dinner Recipes

Dinners are more of a reward for whatever day you have had. It doesn't have to be heavy, but it should be nourishing enough to allow your body to recover from the day thoroughly. Some people would think to skip dinner because they're about to retire for the day. The body performs specific functions during sleep, so you need to supply it with what it needs, so it is renewed for the next morning.

Check out these easy-to-follow recipes:

Sweet Potato and Coconut Curry

Serves: 6

Preparation: 20 minutes

Cooking: 6 hours 30 minutes

Ingredients:

- 250g red cabbage, shredded

- ½ tsp cayenne pepper
- 2 red chilies, seeded and sliced
- 3 garlic cloves, crushed
- 1 small root ginger, peeled
- 400ml coconut milk
- 4 tsp olive oil
- 2 onions, sliced
- 300g passata
- 1 tsp paprika
- 2 tbsp peanut butter
- 2 red peppers, seeded and sliced
- 1 kg sweet potatoes, chopped
- bunch of coriander
- couscous, cooked

Directions:

1. In skillet, heat oil and saute onion and garlic until tender. Add the ginger, paprika, and cayenne. Cook everything for another minute and then put it into the slow cooker.

2. Using the same skillet, heat oil and saute the chili, red cabbage, and red pepper. Cook everything for about 4-5 minutes and then put it into the slow cooker.
3. Using the same skillet, add the remaining oil and fry the sweet potatoes until the edges have browned and then put it into the slow cooker.
4. Cover the contents of the slow cooker with coconut milk and passata. Cover everything and let it cook for about 6-8 hours or until the potatoes are tender.
5. Before finishing, add the peanut butter and season it with salt and pepper. Serve the curry on top of couscous and garnish it with coriander.

Calories	Fat	Carbohydrates	Fiber	Protein	Sodium
434	22g	47g	10g	6g	0.2g

Vegan Shepherd's Pie

Serves: 8

Preparation: 30 minutes

Cooking: 1 hour 20 minutes

Ingredients:

- 4 carrots, cubed
- 4 celery sticks, chopped
- 400g chickpeas
- 3 garlic cloves, crushed
- 2 leeks, chopped
- ½ small pack marjoram or oregano, roughly chopped
- 20ml olive oil
- 2 onions, chopped
- 1 small pack parsley, chopped
- 300g frozen peas
- 30g dried porcini mushrooms, soaked and drained
- 2 tsp smoked paprika

- 1.2kg potatoes
- ½ small pack sage, roughly chopped
- 300g frozen spinach
- 1 butternut squash, peeled and cubed
- ½ small pack thyme, picked
- 2 tbsp tomato puree
- 50ml vegetable oil
- 1 cube vegetable stock
- tomato ketchup (optional)

Directions:
1. Preheat oven to 350°F
2. In a saucepan, bring the unpeeled potatoes to a boil, until the skin separates. Drain and set it aside.
3. In a skillet, heat oil and saute onions, mushrooms, leeks, and carrots. Add vegetable stock and let things simmer.
4. Add garlic, paprika, tomato puree, squash and mixture of herbs. Finally, add the celery and cook everything.

5. Add the chickpeas, including the water in the can, then add the spinach and peas.
6. Peel the potatoes and mash 200g into the stock. Take the rest of the potatoes and combine it with olive oil and parsley.
7. Divide the potato filling into the pie dishes and top them with the chopped potatoes. Pop them into the oven and let it bake for 45 minutes or until the top is golden. Serve with or without ketchup.

Calories	Fat	Carbohydrates	Fiber	Protein	Sodium
348	11g	43g	13g	11g	0.5g

Roast Summer Vegetables and Chickpeas

Serves: 4

Preparation: 20 minutes

Cooking: 50 minutes

Ingredients:

- 1 aubergine, thickly sliced
- 400g can chickpeas
- 1 tbsp coriander seeds
- 1 bunch coriander, roughly chopped
- 3 courgettes, thickly sliced
- 3 garlic cloves, chopped
- 4 tbsp olive oil
- 1 onion, chopped
- 2 red peppers, seeded and chopped
- 2 potatoes, peeled and chopped
- 400g canned tomatoes, chopped

Directions:
1. Preheat oven to 428°F

2. Take a roasting tin and put all the vegetables in it. Season it with coriander seeds, olive oil, salt, and pepper. Pop it into the oven and let it roast for about 45 minutes or until the vegetables turn brown on the edges.
3. Lower the heat and add the chickpeas and tomatoes, then let everything simmer. Drizzle with oil and add coriander just before you take it out of the heat.

Calories	Fat	Carbohydrates	Fiber	Protein	Sodium
327	15g	40g	9g	11g	0.51g

Veggies and Tofu in Peanut Sauce

Serves: 4

Preparation: 10 minutes

Cooking: 10 minutes

Ingredients:

- 1 head broccoli, chopped
- 1 ½ tbsp molasses
- 5 mushroom, sliced
- 1 red bell pepper
- 1 tbsp peanut oil
- ½ cup peanut butter
- 2 tbsp soy sauce
- 1 lb firm tofu, cubed
- 2 tbsp vinegar
- ½ cup hot water
- ground cayenne pepper, to taste

Directions:

1. In a skillet, saute red bell pepper, broccoli, mushroom, and tofu for about 5 minutes
2. Meanwhile in a bowl, combine hot water, peanut butter, soy sauce, vinegar, molasses, and cayenne pepper. Mix it well and pour this over the vegetables in the skillet. Let things simmer until the vegetables are tender.

Calories	Fat	Carbohydrates	Protein	Sodium
442	29.9g	24g	29g	0.641g

Vegan Fajitas

Serves: 6

Preparation: 20 minutes

Cooking: 20 minutes

Ingredients:

- 15 oz black beans
- 1 tsp chili powder
- 8.75 oz whole kernel corn
- ¼ cup, 2 tbsp olive oil
- 1 onion, sliced
- 1 tsp dried oregano
- 1 green bell pepper, julienned
- 1 red bell pepper, julienned
- 4 whole-wheat tortillas
- 1 tsp white sugar
- 2 yellow squash, julienned
- ¼ cup red wine vinegar
- 2 zucchini, julienned
- garlic salt, to taste

- salt and pepper, to taste

Directions:
1. In a bowl, combine vinegar, olive oil, chili powder, oregano, sugar, garlic salt, salt, and pepper. Mix everything well.
2. Add the yellow squash, zucchini, green pepper, red pepper, and onion. Let it marinate in the refrigerator for about 30 minutes. Drain the marinade before cooking.
3. In a skillet, saute the vegetables until they are tender. Add the beans and corn and continue cooking until the vegetables have browned.
4. Arrange the fajitas and stuff the filling into the tortillas to serve

Calories	Fat	Carbohydrates	Protein	Sodium
198	14.4g	17.9g	3g	0.130g

Chapter 8: Vegan Dessert Recipes

There is always room for dessert—and as a vegan, you should still make room for the sweet stuff because it is going to make meals so much more delightful. Do not think that just because you have turned vegan, you cannot enjoy the fun things in life. You are mistaken.

Check out these easy-to-follow recipes:

Vegan Carrot Cake

Serves: 12-15

Preparation: 35 minutes

Cooking: 25 minutes

Ingredients:

- 1 ½ tsp baking powder
- 4 carrots, grated
- 2 tbsp cashew nut butter

- 1 tsp cinnamon
- 4 sachets creamed coconut
- 250ml coconut oil, melted
- 420g plain flour
- 1 tsp ginger
- 1 tbsp lemon juice
- 1 tsp ground nutmeg
- 60ml, 210ml oat milk
- 1 orange, zest only
- 1 ½ tsp bicarbonate of soda
- 300g light brown sugar
- 50g icing sugar
- 1 ½ tsp vanilla essence
- 75g walnuts, chopped
- edible flowers, optional

Directions:

1. In a bowl, combine coconut cream with lemon juice and 2 tbsp hot water. Mix everything well until smooth, then add the cashew butter. Finally, add the icing sugar and once adequately mixed, set it aside in the refrigerator to set.
2. Preheat oven to 350°F. Grease two cake tins with coconut oil.
3. In a bowl, combine sugar and oil then add the milk and vanilla essence. Once mixed, add flour, bicarbonate of soda, baking powder, and orange zest. Lastly, add the carrots and nuts.
4. Divide the batter into the cake tins and pop them into the oven to bake for about 25-30 minutes or until a toothpick comes out cleanly.
5. Pile the cake on top of each other, with a layer of icing in the middle. Then spread the remaining frosting on top of the cake and finish it with a sprinkle of nuts, cinnamon, and edible flowers (if you are using).

Calories	Fat	Carbohydrates	Fiber	Protein	Sodium
501	31g	49g	2g	5g	0.45g

Salted Caramel Biscuit Bar

Makes: 18 pieces

Preparation: 45 minutes

Cooking: 15 minutes

Ingredients:

- 20g ground almonds
- 150g dairy-free dark chocolate
- 3 tbsp, 2 tbsp coconut oil, melted
- 125g Medjool dates pitted
- 50ml maple syrup
- ½ tbsp. almond milk
- 1 ½ tbsp. peanut butter or almond butter
- 80g porridge oats
- pinch of salt

Directions:

1. Preheat oven to 350°F and line a baking dish with parchment paper.

2. In a food processor, combine oats and let it run until flour-like. Add almonds, maple syrup and 3 tbsp coconut oil and mix everything well.
3. Once the batter is formed, roll it and then cut it into rectangular bars, then lay them on the baking sheet. Pop them into the oven and let it bake for about 10 minutes.
4. In the same food processor, combine the dates, peanut butter (or almond butter), coconut oil, and almond milk. Season this with salt and let everything run until it is smooth. One by one, dip the biscuits into the caramel mixture and set it aside.
5. In a heatproof bowl, melt the chocolate over a pan with hot water, making sure the water doesn't get into the chocolate. Dip the caramel dipped biscuits, then lay everything on the tray.
6. Pop the tray into the refrigerator and leave them inside until the chocolate has set.

Calories	Fat	Carbohydrates	Fiber	Protein	Sodium
137	8g	13g	2g	2g	0.1g

Mint-Chip Coconut Milk Ice Cream

Serves: 8

Preparation: 10 minutes

Ingredients:

- 1/3 cup agave syrup
- 3 oz vegan dark chocolate, chopped
- 24 fl oz coconut milk
- 1 tsp peppermint extract

Directions:

1. Chill all the ingredients to make the freezing process much quicker
2. In a blender, combine coconut milk, peppermint extract, and agave syrup. Run it until the mixture is smooth.
3. Following the manufacturer's instructions, transfer the contents to an ice cream maker. Add the chocolate and freeze everything for 2 hours before serving.

Calories	Fat	Carbohydrates	Protein	Sodium
269	22g	19.4g	2.3g	0.012g

Orange Vegan Cake

Serves: 16

Preparation: 15 minutes

Cooking 30 minutes

Ingredients:

- 1 ½ tsp baking soda
- 1 ½ cups all-purpose flour
- 1 orange, peeled
- 1 cup white sugar
- ½ cup vegetable oil
- ¼ tsp salt

Directions:

1. Preheat oven to 375°F, Grease an 8x8 baking pan
2. In a blender, combine orange until you measure 1 cup orange juice
3. In a bowl, combine blended orange juice, sugar, flour, baking soda, vegetable oil, and salt. Whish it well together and pour it into the baking pan.

4. Pop it into the oven and let it bake for 30 minutes or until cooked through and a toothpick comes out cleanly.

Calories	Fat	Carbohydrates	Fiber	Protein	Sodium
157	7g	22.8g	1g	1.3g	0.155g

Vegan Rose Meringues

Serves: 40

Preparation: 30 minutes

Cooking: 1 hour 30 minutes

Ingredients:

- ¾ cup aquafaba (chickpea water)
- ¼ tsp cream of tartar
- ¼ tsp lemon juice
- 1 tsp rose water
- ¾ cup confectioners' sugar

Directions:

1. Preheat oven to 200°F
2. In a large bowl, combine rose water, aquafaba, cream of tartar and lemon juice. Using an electric mixer, blend everything until it is light and fluffy. Add confectioner's sugar, by increments, until you form stiff peaks.

3. Scoop mixture into a piping bag and fit it with a round tip
4. Pipe mounds of the mixture on the baking sheets lined with baking sheets. Pop it into the oven and bake for 1 ½ to 2 hours or until the meringues are dry and firm.

Calories	Fat	Carbohydrates	Protein	Sodium
11	0g	2.4g	0g	0g

Chapter 9: Vegan Soups, Stews and Salads

Soups and salads are great appetizers or side dishes, so it's good to have them either as a small meal or as a filler. Stews, on the other hand, are a specialized type of dish that features a thick and flavorful sauce.

Crunchy Bulgur Salad

Serves: 4

Preparation: 10 minutes

Cooking: 15 minutes

Ingredients:

- 75g whole blanched almonds
- 200g bulgur wheat
- 150g frozen podded edamame (soya) beans
- 1 bunch of mint, finely chopped
- 3 tbsp extra virgin olive oil

- 2 oranges
- 1 bunch of parsley, finely chopped
- 2 romano peppers, seeded and sliced
- 150g radishes, finely sliced

Directions:

1. Cook the bulgur according to package instructions. Set it aside.
2. In a bowl, soak edamame in boiling water for a minute and then drain.
3. In a large bowl, combine the soaked edamame, almonds, radishes, peppers, parsley, and mint.
4. Peel 1 orange and cut them into segments. Add this to the bowl.
5. Juice the other orange and gather it in a small jar and combine it with oil. Season it and then shake it well to let it emulsify. Toss this over your salad.

Calories	Fat	Carbohydrates	Fiber	Protein	Sodium
483	22g	50g	9g	17g	0g

Tomato Soup

Serves: 4

Preparation: 15 minutes

Cooking: 20 minutes

Ingredients:

- 2 bay leaves
- 1 carrot, diced
- 1 celery stick, roughly chopped
- 2 tbsp olive oil
- 1 onion, diced
- 2 tsp tomato puree
- 1 pinch sugar
- 1 ¼ kg tomatoes, cored and quartered
- 1.2 liters vegetable stock
- salt and pepper, to taste
- sour cream (optional)

Directions:

1. In a pan, saute the onion, carrot, and celery. Cook all the vegetables until they are soft and have lost their color. Stir it continuously to avoid it sticking to the bottom of the pan.
2. Add the tomato puree and stir everything until the vegetables turn red.
3. Add the bay leaves and season everything with salt and pepper. Put a lid on the pan to allow the tomatoes to stew until they shrink.
4. Add the vegetable stock and cook until it boils then let it simmer. Remove from heat and let it stand. Remove the bay leaves and let the tomato soup run in the food processor until it is smooth.
5. Return to pan and heat. Season with salt and pepper to taste. You may serve this with chilled sour cream on top.

Calories	Fat	Carbohydrates	Fiber	Protein	Sodium
123	7g	13g	4g	4g	1.08g

Barley and Lentil Stew

Serves: 8

Preparation: 15 minutes

Cooking: 12 hours

Ingredients:

- ¾ cup pearl barley, uncooked
- 1 tsp dried basil
- 3 bay leaves
- 2 tsp garlic, minced
- ¾ cup dry lentils
- ¼ cup dried onion flakes
- 2 cups button mushrooms, sliced
- 1 oz shitake mushrooms, torn
- 2 tsp dried summer savory
- 2 quarts vegetable broth
- salt and pepper, to taste

Directions:

1. In a slow cooker, combine the vegetable broth, shitake mushrooms, button mushrooms, lentils, barley, garlic, onion flakes, summer savory, basil, bay leaves, salt, and pepper.
2. Cover and leave it to cook for about 4 to 6 hours. Remove bay leaves and serve.

Calories	Fat	Carbohydrates	Protein	Sodium
213	1.2g	43.9g	8.4g	0.466g

Spinach and Lentil Soup

Serves: 4

Preparation: 10 minutes

Cooking: 55 minutes

Ingredients:

- 1 tsp ground cumin
- 2 cloves garlic, crushed
- 3 cloves garlic, minced
- ½ cup lentils
- 2 white onions, sliced into rings
- 10 oz spinach
- 1 tbsp vegetable oil
- 2 cups water
- salt and pepper, to taste

1. In a pan, heat oil and saute onions until browned and add garlic, and saute for about a minute.

2. Add the water, and the lentils then bring everything to a boil. Reduce heat and let things simmer until the lentils soften.
3. Add spinach, cumin, and salt. Cover the pan again and let things simmer. Add the crushed garlic and pepper to taste.

Calories	Fat	Carbohydrates	Protein	Sodium
155	4.3g	24g	9.7g	0.639g

Black Bean and Corn Salad

Serves: 6

Preparation: 25 minutes

Ingredients:

- 1 avocado, peeled and diced
- 15 oz black beans
- ½ cup fresh cilantro, chopped
- 1 ½ cup frozen corn kernels
- 1 clove garlic, minced
- 1/3 cup fresh lime juice
- ½ cup olive oil
- 6 green onions, thinly sliced
- 1 red bell pepper, chopped
- 1/8 tsp ground cayenne pepper
- 1 tsp salt

Directions:

1. In a jar with lid, combine olive oil, lime juice, cayenne pepper, garlic, and salt. Cover and shake to combine all the ingredients
2. In a bowl, combine the corn, beans, bell pepper, avocado, tomatoes, cilantro and green onions. Toss everything well and pour the lime dressing over it. Toss the salad to coat the vegetables evenly.

Calories	Fat	Carbohydrates	Protein	Sodium
391	24.5g	35.1g	10.5g	0.830g

Chapter 10: Vegan Snack and Smoothie Recipe

Snacking can be very difficult. In between meals, you will feel slight hunger pangs, and everyone tends to grab a bag of chips or a bar of chocolate. As a transitioning vegan, it will be a challenge, so you have to equip yourself with excellent snacking ideas.

Check out these easy-to-follow recipes:

Strawberry and Oatmeal Smoothie

Serves: 2

Preparation: 10 minutes

Ingredients:

- 1 banana, chunks
- 1 cup almond milk
- ½ cup rolled oats

- 14 strawberries, frozen
- 1 ½ tsp agave nectar (optional)
- ½ tsp vanilla extract (optional)

Directions:

1. In a blender, combine oats, milk, banana, strawberries, vanilla extract and agave nectar and blend it. Run it until it is smooth and serve cold.

Calories	Fat	Carbohydrates	Protein	Sodium
205	2.9g	42.4g	4.2g	0.083mg

Sweet Potato, Chili, and Peanut Butter Quesadillas

Serves: 2

Preparation: 15 minutes

Cooking: 45 minutes

Ingredients:
- 1 ripe avocado, peeled and chopped
- ½ pack coriander, torn
- ½ lime, juice and zest
- 3 tbsp olive oil
- 1 tbsp smoked paprika
- 2 tbsp crunchy peanut butter
- 3 sweet potatoes, thinly sliced
- 4 flour tortillas
- sriracha chili sauce, to taste

Directions:
1. Preheat oven to 400°F

2. In a roasting tin, combine sweet potatoes, 2 tbsp oil, and paprika and pop it in the oven for about 15 minutes or until the potatoes have become crisp.
3. In a bowl, combine avocado, lime zest and. Mash the avocados well, until it is smooth, and add the peanut butter and the remaining olive oil.
4. In a griddle pan, heat the tortillas on either side.
5. To arrange, lay the tortilla and spread the peanut butter mixture then add sweet potatoes and chili sauce. Add the other tortilla and press down to cook it even more. Flip the tortilla and do the same on the other side. Cut it into quarters and serve with lime wedges and crushed avocados.

Calories	Fat	Carbohydrates	Fiber	Protein	Sodium
947	51g	96g	18g	17g	1.7g

Raw Strawberry Jam

Makes: 1 350g jar

Preparation: 15 minutes

Ingredients:

- 2 tbsp chia seeds
- 2 tbsp lemon juice
- 2 tbsp maple syrup
- 400g strawberries, hulled

Directions:

1. In a food processor, blend ¾ strawberries and chop the rest.
2. Add the lemon juice, chia seeds and maple syrup. Stir well and then leave it for an hour to set. Stir it occasionally and wait for it to thicken.
3. Store it in a jar in the refrigerator for 4 days up to a month. Enjoy this on warm toast.

Calories	Fat	Carbohydrates	Fiber	Protein	Sodium
12	0.3g	2g	1g	0.2g	0g

Vegan Cashew Cream Cheese

Makes: 1 400g jar

Preparation: 15 minutes

Ingredients:

- 250g cashews
- 1 juice of lemon
- 2 tbsp nutritional yeast
- 1 tbsp water
- 1 bunch chives (optional)
- ½ tsp salt

Directions:

1. In a bowl, soak the cashews in water for 4 hours or overnight.
2. Drain water from the bowl and transfer the cashews to a food processor. Add lemon juice, nutritional yeast, salt, and water. Let things run until the mixture is smooth.

3. Transfer cream cheese mixture to a bowl and add chives. Store in the refrigerator for an hour and enjoy for as long as 3-4 days.

Calories	Fat	Carbohydrates	Fiber	Protein	Sodium
124	9g	4g	1g	5g	0.3g

Kale and Banana Smoothie

Serves: 1

Preparation: 5 minutes

Ingredients:

- 1 banana
- 1 tbsp flax seeds
- 2 cups kale, chopped
- 1 tsp maple syrup
- ½ cup light unsweetened soy milk

Directions:

1. In a blender, combine banana, flax seeds, kale, soy milk, and maple syrup. Blend it until smooth
2. Serve it over ice, or you can freeze the banana overnight

Calories	Fat	Carbohydrates	Protein	Sodium
311	7.3	56.6g	12.2g	0.110g

Bonus Chapter: 14-Day Vegan Getting Started Plan

Given what you have learned, it is now time for you to apply things and see how well you do. It is not going to be easy, making a switch, especially when it is too drastic. But here is a 14-day plan that you can use as a guide so that you can transition with more ease.

This two-week plan is only a starter, but use it as a template, so that you can fully launch your brand new lifestyle, with much ease.

WEEK 1

DAY	BREAKFAST	LUNCH	DINNER
MONDAY	Vegan Pancakes with Blueberries	Veggie Quesadillas	Ginger Noodles with Mixed Greens Salad
TUESDAY	Cinnamon Apple Oatmeal	Bean and Veggie Toast	Falafel Salad with Tahini Dressing
WEDNESDAY	English Muffin with Peanut Butter and Chia Berry Jam	Potato and Cauliflower Curry	Rainbow Veggie Spring Roll

THURSDAY	Kale and Spinach Smoothie	Stuffed Sweet Potatoes with Hummus	Barbecue-Style Portabello Mushrooms
FRIDAY	Oatmeal with Fresh Fruits and Nuts	Quinoa Pilaf	Chickpea Curry
SATURDAY	Yogurt with Muesli and Mixed Berries	Tomato and Non-Dairy Cheddar Cheese Toast	Mozzarella, Zucchini and Basil Frittata
SUNDAY	Healthy Green Smoothie	Chickpea Salad Roll	Lentil Artichoke Stew

WEEK 2

DAY	BREAKFAST	LUNCH	DINNER
MONDAY	Oatmeal Banana Bites	Balsamic Zucchini Sandwich	Roasted Vegetable Lettuce Wraps
TUESDAY	Strawberry and Oatmeal Breakfast Smoothie	Stir-fry Yam and Bok Choy on Brown Rice	Black Bean Quinoa Bowl
WEDNESDAY	Avocado and Egg on Toast	Edamame Greek Salad	Sweet Potato and Lentil Chilli
THURSDAY	Quinoa Cereal with Almond Milk	Apple and Cheese Pita Pocket	Cashew and Vegetable Stir-fry

FRIDAY	Peanut Butter and Cinnamon Toast	Veggie Fajitas	Vegetarian Pita Pizza
SATURDAY	Loaded Breakfast Burritos	Artichoke and Tomato Gnocchi	Butternut Squash and Black Bean Tostadas
SUNDAY	Cornbread Muffins with Assorted Berries	Chickpea Salad with Roasted Red Pepper Hummus Dressing	Carrot and Red Pepper Soup with Toasted Whole-Wheat Tortillas

Final Words

Thank you again for purchasing this book! I really hope this book is able to help you.

The next step is for you to **join our email newsletter** to receive updates on any upcoming new book releases or promotions. You can sign-up for free and as a bonus, you will also receive our "*7 Fitness Mistakes You Don't Know You're Making*" book! This bonus book breaks down many of the most common fitness mistakes and will demystify many of the complexities and science of getting into shape. Having all this fitness knowledge and science organized into an actionable step-by-step book will help you get started in the right direction in your fitness journey! To join our free email newsletter and grab your free book, please visit the link and signup: **www.hmwpublishing.com/gift**

Finally, if you enjoyed this book, then I would like to ask you for a favor, would you be kind enough to leave a review for this book? It would be greatly appreciated!

Thank you and good luck in your journey!

About the Co-Author

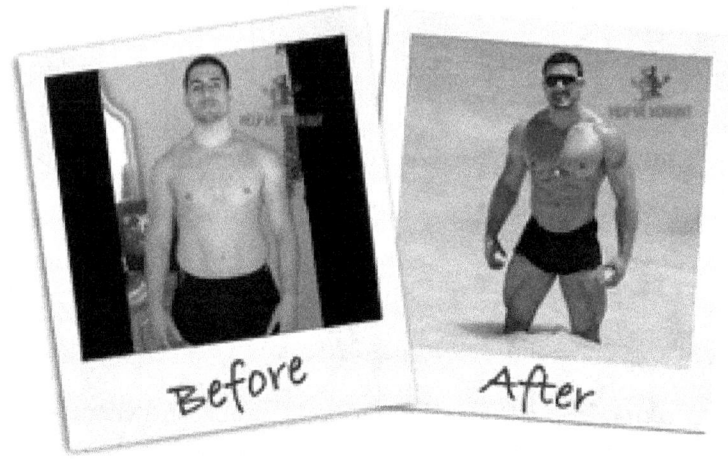

My name is George Kaplo; I'm a certified personal trainer from Montreal, Canada. I'll start off by saying I'm not the biggest guy you will ever meet and this has never really been my goal. In fact, I started working out to overcome my biggest insecurity when I was younger, which was my self-confidence. This was due to my height measuring only 5 foot 5 inches (168cm), it pushed me down to attempt anything I ever wanted to achieve in life. You may be going through some challenges right now, or you may simply want to get fit, and I can certainly relate.

For me personally, I was always kind of interested in the health & fitness world and wanted to gain some muscle due to the numerous bullying in my teenage years about my height and my overweight body. I figured I couldn't do anything about my height, but I sure can do something about how my body looked like. This was the beginning of my transformation journey. I had no idea where to start, but I just got started. I felt worried and afraid at times that other people would make fun of me for doing the exercises the wrong way. I always wished I had a friend that was next to me who was knowledgeable enough to help me get started and "show me the ropes."

After a lot of work, studying and countless trial and errors. Some people began to notice how I was getting more fit and how I was starting to form a keen interest in the topic. This led many friends and new faces to come to me and ask me for fitness advice. At first, it seemed odd when people asked me to help them get in shape. But what kept me going is when they started to see changes in their own body and told me it's the first time that they saw real results!

From there, more people kept coming to me, and it made me realize after so much reading and studying in this field that it did help me but it also allowed me to help others. I'm now a fully certified personal trainer and have trained numerous clients to date who have achieved amazing results.

Today, my brother Alex Kaplo (also a Certified Personal Trainer) and I own & operate this publishing venture, where we bring passionate and expert authors to write about health and fitness topics. We also run an online fitness website "HelpMeWorkout.com" and I would love to connect with by inviting you to visit the website on the following page and signing up to our e-mail newsletter (you will even get a free book).

Last but not least, if you are in the position I was once in and you want some guidance, don't hesitate and ask... I'll be there to help you out!

Your friend and coach,

George Kaplo
Certified Personal Trainer

Get another book for Free

I want to thank you for purchasing this book and offer you another book (just as long and valuable as this book), "Health & Fitness Mistakes You Don't Know You're Making", completely free.

Visit the link below to signup and receive it:

www.hmwpublishing.com/gift

In this book, I will break down the most common health & fitness mistakes, you are probably committing right now, and I will reveal how you can easily get in the best shape of your life!

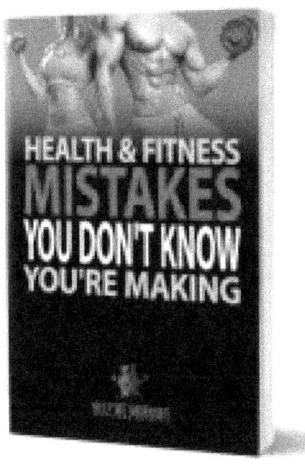

In addition to this valuable gift, you will also have an opportunity to get our new books for free, enter giveaways, and receive other valuable emails from me. Again, visit the link to sign up:

www.hmwpublishing.com/gift

Copyright 2017 by HMW Publishing - All Rights Reserved.

This document by HMW Publishing owned by the A&G Direct Inc company, is geared towards providing exact and reliable information in regards to the topic and issue covered. The publication is sold with the idea that the publisher is not required to render accounting, officially permitted, or otherwise, qualified services. If advice is necessary, legal or professional, a practiced individual in the profession should be ordered.

From a Declaration of Principles which was accepted and approved equally by a Committee of the American Bar Association and a Committee of Publishers and Associations.

In no way is it legal to reproduce, duplicate, or transmit any part of this document in either electronic means or in printed format. Recording of this publication is strictly prohibited, and any storage of this document is not allowed unless with written permission from the publisher. All rights reserved.

The information provided herein is stated to be truthful and consistent, in that any liability, in terms of inattention or otherwise, by any usage or abuse of any policies, processes, or directions contained within is the solitary and utter responsibility of the recipient reader. Under no circumstances will any legal responsibility or blame be held against the publisher for any reparation, damages, or monetary loss due to the information herein, either directly or indirectly.

The information herein is offered for informational purposes solely, and is universal as so. The presentation of the information is without contract or any type of guarantee assurance.

The trademarks that are used are without any consent, and the publication of the trademark is without permission or backing by the trademark owner. All trademarks and brands within this book are for clarifying purposes only and are the owned by the owners themselves, not affiliated with this document.

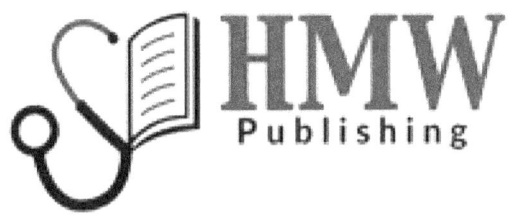

For more great books visit:

HMWPublishing.com

www.ingramcontent.com/pod-product-compliance
Lightning Source LLC
LaVergne TN
LVHW011717060526
838200LV00051B/2933